CW00496759

Keto Diet Cookbook for Your Lunch & Dinner

A Collection of Delicious Keto Diet Recipes for Your Daily Meals

Melody Pope

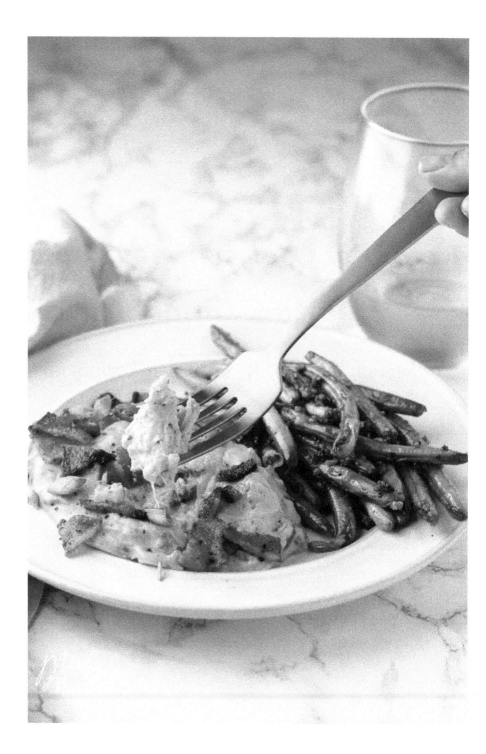

1

© Copyright 2021 - All rights reserved.

The content contained within this book may not be reproduced, duplicated or transmitted without direct written permission from the author or the publisher.

Under no circumstances will any blame or legal responsibility be held against the publisher, or author, for any damages, reparation, or monetary loss due to the information contained within this book. Either directly or indirectly.

Legal Notice:

This book is copyright protected. This book is only for personal use. You cannot amend, distribute, sell, use, quote or paraphrase any part, or the content within this book, without the consent of the author or publisher.

Disclaimer Notice:

Please note the information contained within this document is for educational and entertainment purposes only. All effort has been executed to present accurate, up to date, and reliable, complete information. No warranties of any kind are declared or implied. Readers acknowledge that the author is not engaging in the rendering of legal, financial, medical or professional advice. The content within this book has been derived from various sources. Please consult a licensed professional before attempting any techniques outlined in this book.

By reading this document, the reader agrees that under no circumstances is the author responsible for any losses, direct or indirect, which are incurred as a result of the use of information contained within this document, including, but not limited to, — errors, omissions, or inaccuracies.

Table of Contents

Sweet & Tangy Beef Shoulder

Preparation Time: 15 minutes

Cooking Time: 9 hours 10 minutes

Servings: 14

Ingredients:

- ¼ cup unsalted butter
- 8 pounds grass-fed chuck shoulder roast
- Salt
- Ground black pepper
- 1 yellow onion, chopped
- 4 garlic cloves, minced
- 1 tablespoon Dijon mustard
- 2 tablespoons vinegar
- 2 tablespoons fresh lemon juice
- 3-4 drops liquid stevia

Directions:

1. Dissolve the butter in a large skillet over medium-high heat and cook beef with salt and black pepper for about 1-2 minutes per side.

2. Transfer the beef into a large crockpot. In the same skillet, add onion and sauté for about 2-3 minutes. Place onion evenly over beef.

3. In a bowl, mix the remaining ingredients. Pour the sauce evenly over beef. Set the crockpot on low and cook, covered, for about 9 hours.

4. Uncover the crockpot and transfer the beef to a cutting board. Transfer the sauce into a small pan over medium-high heat and cook for about 5 minutes or until desired thickness.

5. Cut beef shoulder into desired sized slices. Pour sauce over beef slices and serve.

Nutrition:

- Calories: 516
- Carbohydrates: 1.1g
- Protein: 48.4g
- Fat: 33.1g

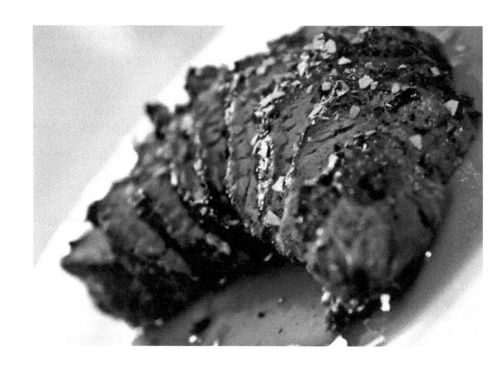

Succulent Beef Pot Roast

Preparation Time : 15 minutes

Cooking Time: 8 hours

Servings: 6

Ingredients:

- 2 pounds grass-fed beef pot roast
- 1 yellow onion, sliced
- 2 garlic cloves, minced
- 2 jalapeño peppers, minced
- 1 tablespoon fresh rosemary, minced
- ¼ cup fresh lemon juice
- ½ cup homemade beef broth
- 1 teaspoon ground cumin
- Salt
- Ground black pepper

Directions:

1. Put grass-fed beef pot roast, and other fixing in a large crockpot and stir to combine. Cook on low within 6-8 hours.

2. Uncover the crockpot and transfer the beef roast to a cutting board. Cut beef roast into desired sized slices and serve.

Nutrition:

- Calories: 298
- Carbohydrates: 2.6g
- Protein: 46.7g
- Fat: 9.9g

Divine Beef Shanks

Preparation Time: 15 minutes

Cooking Time: 8 hours 10 minutes

Servings: 10

Ingredients:

- 3 tablespoons unsalted butter
- 5 (1-pound) grass-fed beef shanks
- Salt
- Ground black pepper
- 1 large yellow onion, chopped
- 10 garlic cloves, minced
- 2 tablespoons sugar-free tomato paste
- 4 fresh rosemary sprigs
- 4 fresh thyme sprigs
- 2 cups homemade beef broth

Directions:

1. Dissolve the butter over medium-high heat in a large skillet and cook beef shanks with salt and black pepper for about 4-5 minutes per side.

2. Transfer the beef shanks to a large crockpot. In the same skillet, sauté onion for about 3-4 minutes. Add garlic and sauté within 1 minute.

3. Place onion mixture over beef shanks and cover evenly with tomato paste. With a kitchen string, tie the herbs sprigs.

4. Arrange tied sprigs over tomato paste and pour the broth on top evenly. Set the crockpot on low and cook, covered, for about 8 hours. Serve hot.

Nutrition:

- Calories: 513
- Carbohydrates: 3.2g
- Protein: 77.9g
- Fat: 18.9g

Family Dinner Beef Brisket

Preparation Time: 15 minutes

Cooking Time: 6 hours

Servings: 12

Ingredients:

- 1 large yellow onion, sliced
- 3 garlic cloves, chopped
- 1 (4-pound) grass-fed beef brisket
- ½ teaspoon red pepper flakes, crushed
- ½ teaspoon smoked paprika
- ½ teaspoon ground cumin
- Salt
- Ground black pepper
- 2 cups homemade beef broth

Directions:

1. In a large crockpot, put all the fixing and stir to combine. Cook on low, covered, within 6 hours. Uncover the crockpot and transfer the beef brisket onto a cutting board. Cut beef brisket into desired sized slices and serve.

Nutrition:

- Calories: 353

- Carbohydrates: 2g
- Protein: 56.3g
- Fat: 11.6g

Italian Beef Stroganoff

Preparation Time: 15 minutes

Cooking Time: 8 hours

Servings: 8

Ingredients:

- 4 pounds grass-fed beef short ribs
- ½ teaspoon red pepper flakes, crushed
- Salt
- Ground black pepper
- 1 cup button mushrooms, sliced
- 1½ cups tomatoes, chopped finely
- ½ cup onion, chopped
- 4 garlic cloves, minced
- 2 tablespoons fresh basil leaves, chopped
- 2 cups homemade beef broth
- ½ cup dry white wine

Directions:

1. In a large crockpot, put all the listed fixing, then stir. Set the crockpot on low and cook, covered, for about 4-6 hours. Serve hot.

Nutrition:

- Calories: 500
- Carbohydrates: 3.5g
- Protein: 67.5g
- Fat: 20.9g

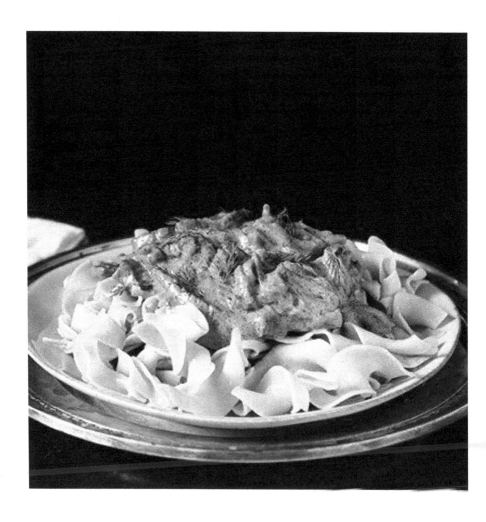

Energizing Beef Casserole

Preparation Time: 20 minutes

Cooking Time: 9 hours

Servings: 5

Ingredients:

- 1-pound grass-fed beef steak, cut into thin strips
- Salt
- Ground black pepper
- 1 small yellow onion, sliced
- 1 cup tomatoes, chopped
- 1 cup fresh mushrooms, sliced
- 1¼ cups fresh green beans
- ½ cup homemade beef broth

Directions:

1. In a large crockpot, put all the above fixing and stir to combine. Set the crockpot on low and cook, covered, for about 8 hours. Serve hot.

Nutrition:

- Calories: 196
- Carbohydrates: 5.2g
- Protein: 29.4g

- Fat: 5.9g

North American Pork Ribs

Preparation Time: 20 minutes

Cooking Time: 10 hours

Servings: 6

Ingredients:

- 3 pounds pork ribs
- 1 small yellow onion, chopped
- 2 garlic cloves, minced
- 1 cup baby carrots, peeled and chopped
- ½ cup homemade chicken broth
- ¼ cup coconut aminos
- 1 tablespoon olive oil
- Salt
- Ground black pepper

Directions:

1. In a large crockpot, add all ingredients and stir to combine. Set the crockpot on low and cook, covered, within 8-10 hours. Serve hot.

Nutrition:

- Calories: 506
- Carbohydrates: 5.8g

- Protein: 45.9g
- Fat: 32g

Simply Delicious Pork Chops

Preparation Time: 15 minutes

Cooking Time: 5 hours 5 minutes

Servings: 5

Ingredients:

- 1 tablespoon coconut oil
- 2 garlic cloves, minced
- 5 (4-ounce) boneless pork chops
- Salt
- Ground black pepper
- 1 large zucchini, cubed
- 2 lemons, sliced
- 1 teaspoon red pepper flakes, crushed

Directions:

1. In a large skillet, heat-up oil on medium-high heat and sauté garlic for about 1 minute. Add chops and cook for 1-2 minutes per side.

2. Transfer the chops mixture into a crockpot. Place cubed zucchini over chops evenly, followed by lemon slices.

3. Sprinkle with red pepper flakes, salt, and black pepper. Set the crockpot on High and cook, covered, for about 5 hours. Serve hot

Nutrition:

- Calories: 206
- Carbohydrates: 4.9g
- Protein: 30.8g
- Fat: 7g

Fall-of-the-Bone Pork Shoulder

Preparation Time: 15 minutes

Cooking Time: 8 hours 10 minutes

Servings: 8

Ingredients:

- 2 tablespoons olive oil
- 3 pounds of pork shoulder
- Salt
- Ground black pepper
- 1 medium yellow onion, chopped
- 1 celery stalk, chopped
- 2 garlic cloves, minced
- 2 cups fresh tomatoes, chopped finely
- ½ cup homemade chicken broth
- 2 tablespoons fresh lemon juice

Directions:

1. In a large skillet, heat-up oil on medium-high heat and cook pork shoulder with salt and black pepper for about 4-5 minutes per side.

2. Transfer pork shoulder to a crockpot and top with onion, celery, garlic, and tomatoes. Pour broth and lemon juice on top.

3. Set the crockpot on low and cook, covered, for about 8 hours. Uncover the crockpot and transfer the pork shoulder onto a cutting board. Cut pork shoulder into desired sized slices and serve.

Nutrition:

- Calories: 545
- Carbohydrates: 3.5g
- Protein: 40.5g
- Fat: 40.1g

Christmas Dinner Pork Roast

Preparation Time: 15 minutes

Cooking Time: 8 hours

Servings: 10

Ingredients:

- 4 pounds boneless pork roast
- 1 teaspoon dried rosemary, crushed
- 1 teaspoon dried thyme, crushed
- 1 teaspoon cayenne pepper
- ½ teaspoon smoked paprika
- Salt
- Ground black pepper
- 1 medium yellow onion, sliced thinly and divided
- 1 cup hot homemade chicken broth

Directions:

1. Rub the pork with herbs and spices generously. At the bottom of a large crockpot, place half the onion and top with pork roast, followed by the remaining onion.

2. Pour broth on top. Set the crockpot on low and cook, covered, for about 6-8 hours. Uncover the crockpot and

transfer the pork roast onto a cutting board. Cut pork roast into desired sized slices and serve.

Nutrition:

- Calories: 269
- Carbohydrates: 1.4g
- Protein: 48.1g
- Fat: 17.5g

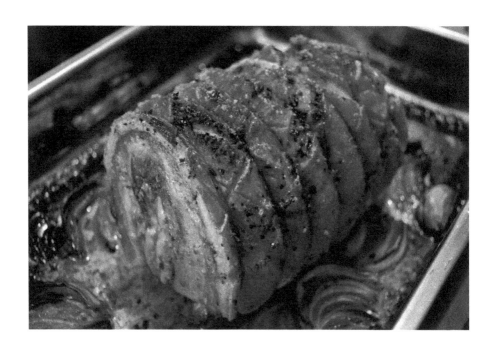

Asian Style Pork Butt

Preparation Time: 15 minutes

Cooking Time : 8 hours

Servings: 8

Ingredients:

- 1 medium onion, sliced thinly
- 4 garlic cloves, minced
- 3 tablespoons lemongrass, minced
- 1 tablespoon vinegar
- 3 tablespoons olive oil
- Salt
- Ground black pepper
- 3 pounds pork butt, trimmed
- 1 cup unsweetened coconut milk

Directions:

1. In a large bowl, add garlic, lemongrass, vinegar, oil, and seasoning. Rub the pork butt with garlic mixture evenly.

2. In a large crockpot, place the onion slices and top with pork butt. Cover the crockpot and set aside to marinate for at least 8 hours.

3. Uncover the crockpot and pour coconut milk on top. Set the crockpot on low and cook, covered, for about 8 hours.

4. Uncover the crockpot and transfer the pork butt onto a cutting board. Cut pork butt into desired sized slices and serve.

Nutrition:

- Calories: 445
- Carbohydrates: 3.9g
- Protein: 53.9g
- Fat: 23.8g

Meaty Pie

Preparation time: 15 minutes

Cooking time: 6 hours & 30 minutes

Servings: 6

Ingredients:

- 1 ½ pounds ground beef
- 1 egg
- ½ cup almonds ground finely into a flour
- ½ cup Parmesan cheese, freshly grated
- ½ cup green bell pepper, diced
- ½ cup onion, diced
- 1 teaspoon salt
- 1 teaspoon black pepper
- 1 tablespoon fresh oregano
- 2 cups tomatoes, chopped
- 2 garlic cloves, crushed and minced
- ½ cup fresh basil, chopped
- 1 cup fresh Mozzarella, sliced

Directions:

1. Mix the ground beef, egg, almonds, Parmesan cheese, green bell pepper, and onion in a bowl. Flavor the mixture with salt, black pepper, plus oregano. Mix well.

2. Take the meat mixture and press it firmly into the bottom of the slow cooker. Place the tomatoes, garlic, and basil in a blender and puree. Pour the tomato mixture over the meat. Cover and cook on low within 6 hours.

3. Remove the lid and arrange the mozzarella cheese slices over the top. Replace the cover and cook within 30 minutes before serving.

Nutrition:

- Calories: 406.7
- Fat: 31.7g
- Carbs: 7.2g
- Protein: 23.7g

Mexican Meatloaf

Preparation time: 15 minutes

Cooking time: 7 hours

Servings: 6

Ingredients:

- 1 ½ pounds ground beef
- 1 egg
- 1 cup añejo cheese, grated
- 1 cup onion, diced
- 2 tablespoons jalapeño pepper, diced
- ¼ cup fresh cilantro, chopped
- 2 teaspoons chili powder
- 1 teaspoon ground cumin
- 1 teaspoon salt
- 1 teaspoon black pepper
- 1 cup roasted tomatoes, chopped
- ½ cup Mexican crema
- 1 avocado, sliced

Directions:

1. Mix the ground beef, egg, añejo cheese, onion, and jalapeño pepper in a bowl. Season the mixture with the

cilantro, chili powder, cumin, salt, and black pepper. Mix well.

2. Line a slow cooker with aluminum foil for easier removal, if desired. Take the meat mixture and either form it into a loaf, place it in the slow cooker, or press the meat mixture into the slow cooker's bottom.

3. Add the tomatoes on top of the meatloaf. Cover and cook on low for 7 hours, or until cooked through. Serve garnished with a dollop of Mexican crema and sliced avocado.

Nutrition:

- Calories: 545.2
- Fat: 45.6g
- Carbs: 8.3g
- Protein: 26.7g

Whiskey Blues Steak

Preparation time: 15 minutes

Cooking time: 6 hours

Servings: 6

Ingredients:

- 1 ½ pound beef steak
- 1 teaspoon salt
- 2 teaspoons coarsely ground black pepper
- 3 cups zucchini, sliced thick
- ¼ cup butter
- 1 cup onions, sliced
- ¼ cup whiskey
- 2 garlic cloves, crushed and minced
- ½ cup blue cheese, crumbled

Directions:

1. Flavor the steak with salt plus black pepper. Place the sliced zucchini in the bottom of the slow cooker.

2. Melt the butter in a skillet over medium-high heat. Add the steaks to the skillet and brown on both sides, approximately 2-4 minutes.

3. Remove the steaks from the skillet and place them in the slow cooker. Add the onions to the skillet and sauté until crisp-tender, approximately 3-4 minutes.

4. Add the whiskey and cook until reduced, 1-2 minutes, scraping the bottom of the skillet. Put the onions back in the slow cooker and sprinkle in the garlic.

5. Cover and cook on low within 6 hours, or until the steaks are cooked to the desired doneness and are tender. Serve the steaks garnished with blue cheese.

Nutrition:

- Calories: 305
- Fat: 15.4g
- Carbs: 6.1g
- Protein: 29.2g

Philly Cheese Steak

Preparation time: 15 minutes

Cooking time: 4 hours & 30 minutes

Servings: 6

Ingredients:

- 1 cup green bell pepper, sliced
- 1 cup onion, sliced
- ¼ cup of butter melted
- 1 ½ pound beef steak, sliced thin
- 4 garlic cloves, crushed and minced
- ¼ cup Worcestershire sauce
- ¼ cup beef stock
- ¼ cup of soy sauce
- 1 teaspoon salt
- 1 teaspoon black pepper
- 1 teaspoon paprika
- 1 cup Swiss cheese, shredded
- Bibb lettuce leaves or approved keto bread for serving (optional)

Directions:

1. Place the green bell pepper and the onion in a slow cooker. Pour in the butter and toss to coat. Add the sliced beef steak into the slow cooker.

2. In a bowl, combine the garlic, Worcestershire sauce, beef stock, soy sauce, salt, black pepper, and paprika. Mix well and pour the liquid into the slow cooker.

3. Cook on high within 4 hours. Remove the lid and sprinkle in the Swiss cheese. Replace the cover, turn the heat to low, and cook an additional 30 minutes before serving.

Nutrition:

- Calories: 312.6
- Fat: 17.1g
- Carbs: 6.6g
- Protein: 32.2g

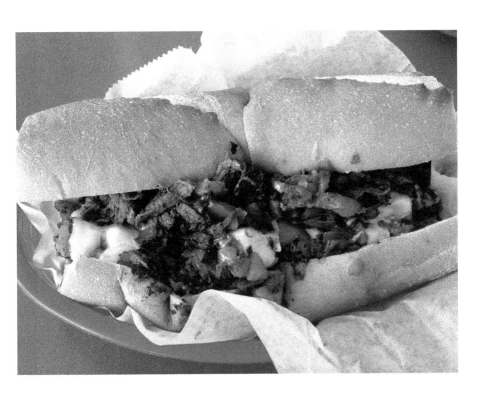

Steak Stuffed Peppers

Preparation time: 15 minutes

Cooking time : 4 hours

Servings: 4

Ingredients:

- 4 red bell peppers
- 2 tablespoons butter
- 1-pound beef steak, sliced thin
- 1 teaspoon salt
- 1 teaspoon black pepper
- 1 tablespoon fresh rosemary, finely chopped
- ¼ cup fresh basil, chopped
- 4 garlic cloves, crushed and minced
- 1 cup tomatoes, chopped
- ½ cup onion, diced
- ½ cup celery, diced
- ½ cup walnuts, chopped
- ½ cup Stilton cheese, crumbled
- 1 cup beef stock or water

Directions:

1. Slice the bell pepper's tops off and scoop the seeds out. Dissolve the butter over medium heat in a skillet. Place the steak in the skillet and cook for 1-2 minutes.

2. Season the steak with salt, black pepper, rosemary, basil, and garlic. Add the tomatoes and cook for an additional 2-3 minutes. Remove, then allow it to cool enough to handle.

3. Combine the steak with the onion, celery, walnuts, and Stilton cheese. Scoop equal amounts of the steak mixture into each of the peppers. Pour the beef stock or water into the slow cooker.

4. Replace the tops on the peppers and arrange them in the slow cooker. Cover and cook on high within 4 hours.

Nutrition:

- Calories: 397
- Fat: 26.4g
- Carbs: 11.0g
- Protein: 33.0g

Spicy Citrus Meatballs

Preparation time: 15 minutes

Cooking time: 8 hours

Servings: 6

Ingredients:

- 1 ½ pounds ground beef
- 1 egg
- 1 tablespoon Worcestershire sauce
- 1 tablespoon garlic chili sauce
- ½ cup onion, diced
- 1 cup zucchini, shredded
- 2 tablespoons olive oil
- 3 cups green beans, trimmed
- 1 cup beef stock
- 1 tablespoon crushed red pepper flakes
- ¼ cup of soy sauce
- 1 teaspoon orange extract
- 1 teaspoon black pepper

Directions:

1. Mix the ground beef, egg, Worcestershire sauce, garlic chili sauce, onion, and zucchini in a bowl. Take spoonsful

of the meat mixture and form them into golf ball-sized meatballs.

2. Pour the olive oil into a skillet over medium heat. Place the meatballs in the skillet and cook just until browned on all sides. Place the green beans in the slow cooker.

3. Transfer the meatballs from the skillet to the slow cooker. Combine the beef stock, crushed red pepper flakes, soy sauce, orange extract, and black pepper, then put into the slow cooker. Cover and cook on low within 8 hours.

Nutrition:
- Calories: 434.6
- Fat: 35.8g
- Carbs: 6.5g
- Protein: 21.7g

Swedish Broccoli and Meatballs

Preparation time: 15 minutes

Cooking time: 7 hours & 30 minutes

Servings: 6

Ingredients:

- 1-pound ground beef
- ½ cup onion, diced
- ½ cup celery, diced
- 2 garlic cloves, crushed and minced
- 1 cup heavy cream, divided
- ½ cup Parmesan cheese, freshly grated
- 1 tablespoon olive oil
- 4 cups broccoli florets
- 1 teaspoon salt
- 1 teaspoon black pepper
- ¼ cup butter, melted
- ½ cup sour cream
- 1 tablespoon fresh chives
- 1 tablespoon fresh thyme

Directions:

1. Mix the ground beef, onion, celery, garlic, ¼ cup of the heavy cream, and the Parmesan cheese in a bowl.

2. Get a spoonful of it, then form them into meatballs measuring approximately one inch in diameter. Heat-up olive oil in a skillet over medium heat.

3. Place the meatballs in the skillet and cook just until browned. Place the broccoli, seasoned with salt and black pepper, in the slow cooker, followed by the butter. Toss to coat.

4. Transfer the meatballs from the skillet to the slow cooker. Cover and cook on low for 7 hours. Combine the remaining heavy cream, sour cream, chives, and thyme.

5. Lift the lid off the slow cooker, add the cream mixture, and stir. Replace the lid and cook an additional 30 minutes before serving.

Nutrition:

- Calories: 561.2
- Fat: 51.4g
- Carbs: 6.8g
- Protein: 19.5g

Balsamic Dijon Short Ribs

Preparation time: 15 minutes

Cooking time: 8 hours

Servings: 6

Ingredients:

- 2 pounds beef short ribs
- 1 teaspoon salt
- 1 teaspoon black pepper
- 2 tablespoons olive oil
- 2 cups Napa cabbage, shredded
- ¼ cup balsamic vinegar
- ¼ cup Dijon mustard
- ½ cup beef stock
- 1 tablespoon fresh thyme
- 2 garlic cloves, crushed and minced

Directions:

1. Flavor the ribs with salt plus black pepper. Heat-up olive oil in a skillet over medium heat. Place the ribs in the skillet and cook for 1-2 minutes per side.

2. Spread the cabbage in the bottom of the slow cooker. Transfer the ribs from the skillet to the slow cooker.

3. Combine the balsamic vinegar, Dijon mustard, beef stock, thyme, garlic, and mix well. Pour the mixture over the ribs. Cover and cook on low within 8 hours.

Nutrition:

- Calories: 282.1
- Fat: 15.4g
- Carbs: 1.8g
- Protein: 30.4g

Slow Cooker Winter Veggies

Preparation time: 15 minutes

Cooking time: 3 hours

Servings: 4

Ingredients:

- 2 cups sliced leeks
- 1 cup carrots, sliced
- 1 ½ cups red onion, diced
- 2 cups butternut squash, diced
- 1 cup celery, sliced
- ½ cup of balsamic vinegar
- ½ cup olive oil
- 2 tablespoons fresh mint, chopped
- 1 tablespoon fresh dill, chopped

Directions:

1. Combine the vegetables in a large bowl. Combine the olive oil and balsamic in another bowl. Stir in the mint and dill.

2. Place vegetables in your slow cooker and cover with the marinade. Stir until the vegetables are cooked entirely. Cook on high for three hours, stirring every hour.

Nutrition:

- Calories: 233
- Fat: 18g
- Protein: 3g
- Carbs: 18g

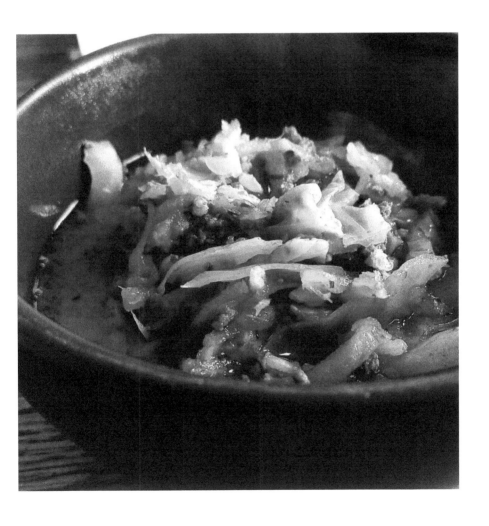

Cauliflower Breakfast Casserole

Preparation time: 15 minutes

Cooking time: 5 hours

Servings: 4

Ingredients:

- 1 egg
- ½ cup milk
- ½ teaspoon dry mustard
- 1 teaspoon salt
- ½ teaspoon pepper
- 1 head cauliflower, shredded
- 1 onion, diced
- 2 5-ounce packages vegetarian sausage crumbles
- 2 cups of shredded cheddar cheese

Directions:

1. Beat the eggs, milk, dry mustard, and salt and pepper. Place one-third of the shredded cauliflower at the bottom of the slow cooker, then add one-third of the onion. Sprinkle with salt and pepper.

2. Add one-third of the vegetarian sausage and cheddar cheese. Repeat these two more times. Pour the egg

mixture over everything, cover, and cook on low for 5 hours or until the top is browned.

Nutrition:

- Calories: 215
- Fat: 18g
- Protein: 3g
- Carbs: 18g

Mexican Cauliflower Rice

Preparation time: 15 minutes

Cooking time: 4 hours

Servings: 4

Ingredients:

- 1-pound cauliflower, cut into medium-sized florets
- 1 cup tomato sauce
- ½ cup of water
- 1 tablespoon tomato paste
- 1 medium white onion, diced
- 2 red bell peppers, diced
- 2 jalapeno peppers, seeded and diced
- 1 tablespoon garlic powder
- 2 teaspoons chipotle powder
- 2 teaspoons cumin
- 1 teaspoon oregano
- 1 teaspoon pepper

Directions:

1. Put the water, tomato sauce, plus tomato paste in the slow cooker. Blend. Add the spices and stir. Add the onion and peppers, and stir. Add the cauliflower and coat the cauliflower with the liquid.

2. Cook on low for 5 hours. Once it is done, use a potato masher or blunt object to mash it until you get a rice-like consistency.

3. Stir it well and drain any extra liquid. If you store this in the fridge, note that the cauliflower will absorb more liquid as it sits.

Nutrition:

- Calories: 205
- Fat: 18g
- Protein: 3g
- Carbs: 18g

Vegetable Ratatouille

Preparation time: 15 minutes

Cooking time: 4 hours

Servings: 6

Ingredients:

- 1 large red bell pepper, slice into squares
- 1 large eggplant, diced
- 2 large zucchinis, diced
- 1 large yellow onion, diced
- 3-2 garlic cloves, finely chopped
- 1 25-ounce jar of tomato sauce or pasta sauce
- Pinch of fresh basil

Directions:

1. Place all ingredients in the crockpot and cover with the sauce. Cook on high for 4 hours. Serve with freshly chopped basil

Nutrition:

- Calories: 215
- Fat: 18g
- Protein: 3g
- Carbs: 8g

Crockpot Parmesan Lemon Cauliflower

Preparation time: 15 minutes

Cooking time: 2 hours

Servings: 4

Ingredients :

- 1-pound cauliflower
- 2 tablespoons butter
- 2 tablespoon fresh sage or powdered
- 2 tablespoons lemon juice
- 1 cup parmesan cheese
- Parsley to garnish

Directions:

1. Place all the fixing in a bowl and thoroughly cover the cauliflower with the butter, sage, and lemon. Cook on low for 2 hours.

2. Once done, add parmesan cheese and a bit more lemon and let it steam for 10 minutes. Serve with a topping of fresh parsley.

Nutrition:

- Calories: 180
- Fat: 18g

- Protein: 3g
- Carbs: 18g

Garlic Herb Mushrooms

Preparation time: 15 minutes

Cooking time: 4 hours

Servings: 4

Ingredients:

- ¼ teaspoon thyme
- 2 bay leaves
- 1 cup vegetable broth
- ½ cup half and half
- 2 tablespoons butter
- 2 tablespoons fresh parsley, chopped
- Salt and pepper, to taste

Directions:

1. Place all of the ingredients save for the butter and the half and half in the slow cooker and put on low for 3 hours. Once done, add the butter and half for the last 15 minutes. Garnish with parsley and enjoy.

Nutrition:

- Calories: 175
- Fat: 18g
- Protein: 3g

- Carbs: 18g

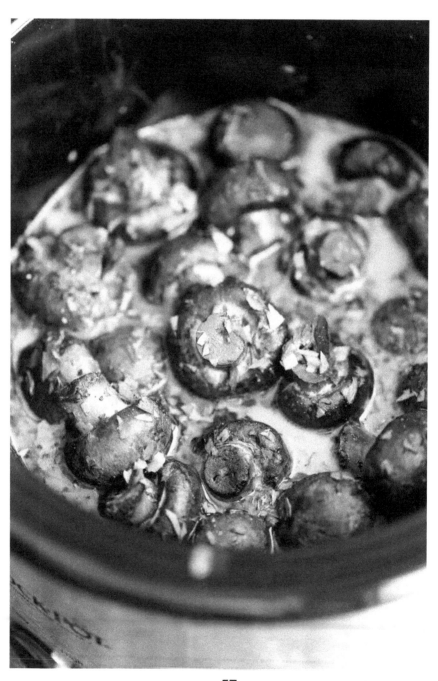

Sticky Sesame Cauliflower Slow Cooker Bites

Preparation time: 15 minutes

Cooking time: 2 hours

Servings: 4

Ingredients:

- 1-pound cauliflower
- ½ teaspoon paprika
- ½ teaspoon ground cumin
- 1 teaspoon garlic powder
- 1 teaspoon sesame oil
- 1/3 cup honey
- 2 tablespoons apple cider vinegar
- 1 teaspoon sweet chili sauce
- 3 garlic cloves, minced
- ¼ cup of water
- 1 tablespoon arrowroot powder or cornstarch
- 1 cup green onions to garnish
- Sesame seeds to garnish

Directions:

1. Place all spices, minus the green onions and sesame seeds, in a bowl, and cover the cauliflower thoroughly with the mixture. Place the cauliflower into the slow cooker.

2. Add the rest of the ingredients and cover. Cook on low for 2 hours. The sauce will thicken with the cornstarch or arrowroot powder. When done, remove each bite and garnish with toasted sesame seeds and green onion slices on top.

Nutrition:

- Calories: 240
- Fat: 7g
- Protein: 3g
- Carbs: 18g

Crockpot Cauliflower Mac and Cheese

Preparation time: 15 minutes

Cooking time: 4 hours

Servings : 4

Ingredients:

- 1-pound cauliflower
- 2 cups shredded cheddar cheese
- 2 ½ cups milk
- 1 12-ounce can evaporate milk
- ½ tablespoon mustard

Directions:

1. Place all of the fixings above in the slow cooker and put on low for 3 hours until most of the liquid has been absorbed.

2. Sprinkle some extra cheese on top and cook for 15 minutes until it has melted and the rest of the liquid is absorbed. Garnish with some parsley and even shredded parmesan cheese.

Nutrition:

- Calories: 215
- Fat: 4g

- Protein: 3g
- Carbs: 18g

Crockpot Vegetable Lasagna

Preparation time: 15 minutes

Cooking time: 2 hours

Servings: 4

Ingredients:

- 2 medium zucchinis
- 1 medium eggplant
- 2 cups tomato-based pasta sauce
- 1 red onion, diced
- 1 red bell pepper, diced
- 16 ounces low fat cottage cheese
- 2 large eggs
- 8 ounces shredded Mozzarella
- 2 tablespoons basil, chopped
- 2 tablespoons parmesan cheese, for garnish

Directions:

1. Slice eggplant plus zucchini lengthwise into thin strips, approximately ¼ inch thick so that they resemble the shape of lasagna noodles. Spread them out over a layer of paper towels and toss with salt.

2. Let stand for 15 minutes to absorb the salt. It helps the vegetables to absorb the liquid. Lightly coat the bottom of your crockpot and spread ½ cup of tomato sauce along the bottom.

3. In a separate bowl, beat the eggs and cottage cheese. Create a layer of "noodles," then 1/3 of the cottage cheese mixture, 1/3 of the bell peppers and onions, and 1/3 of the mozzarella and tomato sauce.

4. Put down another layer of "noodles," then repeat. Finish with the third layer of "noodles." Cook on high for 2 hours, until the eggplant is tender. Slice and scoop out portions as desired, then garnish with herbs and cheese.

Nutrition:

- Calories: 213
- Fat: 9g
- Protein: 3g
- Carbs: 18g

Tasty Tagine Five a Day

Preparation time: 15 minutes

Cooking time: 8 hours

Servings: 6

Ingredients:

- 4 tablespoons of olive oil
- 1 sliced red onion
- 2 cloves of crushed garlic
- 500 grams of aubergine in 1 cm-thick slice, cut lengthways
- 300 grams of quartered ripe tomatoes
- 1 small sliced fennel bulb
- 50 grams of sundried tomatoes
- 1 teaspoon of coriander seeds

For the dressing:

- 100 grams of feta cheese, and extra for topping
- 50 grams of toasted almond flakes

Directions:

1. Put two tbsp of olive oil into the slow cooker and add the crushed garlic and the onions. Brush the aubergines with

the remaining olive oil and place them on top of the onions and garlic.

2. Arrange the sundried tomatoes, fennel slices, and the tomatoes around the aubergines. Flavor it with salt plus pepper and pour the coriander seeds over the top. Cook for 6-8 hours on low.

3. Place the dressing ingredients into a food processor and work until smooth. Spoon the vegetables onto serving dishes, drizzle the dressing over the top and crumble the feta cheese on top.

Nutrition:

- Calories: 289
- Fat: 20g
- Carbs: 11g
- Protein: 8g

Baked Mushrooms with Pesto & Ricotta

Preparation time: 15 minutes

Cooking time: 6 hours

Servings: 4

Ingredients:

- 5 tablespoons of olive oil, extra virgin
- 16 large chestnut mushrooms
- A 250-gram tub of ricotta
- 2 tablespoons of pesto
- 2 finely chopped cloves of garlic
- 25 grams of freshly grated parmesan cheese
- 2 tablespoons of fresh, chopped parsley

Directions:

1. Slice the mushroom stems level with the caps. In a small bowl, combine the garlic, pesto, and ricotta, and spoon into the mushroom heads.

2. Place the mushroom caps in a slow cooker and cook on low for 4-6 hours. In the last half-hour, sprinkle the parmesan cheese over the top of the mushrooms. Serve topped with the fresh parsley.

Nutrition:

- Calories: 400
- Fat: 34g
- Carbohydrates: 2g
- Protein: 19g

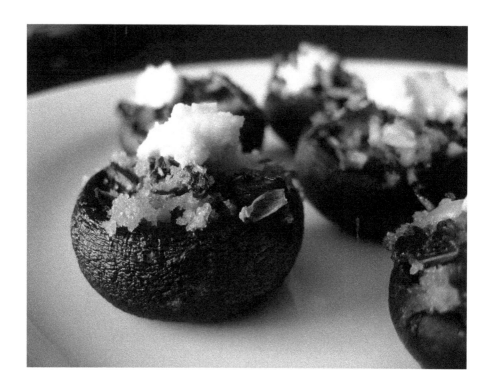

Dal with Crispy Onions

Preparation time: 15 minutes

Cooking time: 6 hours

Servings: 4

Ingredients:

- 250 grams of black urad beans
- 100 grams of ghee or butter
- 2 large onions thinly sliced
- 3 cloves of crushed garlic
- 1 piece of ginger, thumb-sized and finely chopped
- 2 teaspoons of ground cumin
- 2 teaspoons of ground coriander
- 1 teaspoon of ground turmeric
- 1 teaspoon of paprika
- ¼ teaspoon of chili powder
- A small bunch of fresh coriander, reserve the leaves and finely chop the stems
- 400 grams of passata
- 1 red chili, pierced with the tip of a knife
- 50 ml of double cream

For serving:

- Baked sweet potato

- Naan bread
- Cooked rice
- Coriander
- Sliced red chili
- Lime wedges
- Yogurt, cream, or swirl
- Indian chutney or pickle
- Crispy salad onions

Directions:

1. Soak the beans within 4 hours or overnight in cold water. Dissolve the ghee or butter in a large saucepan, then add the ginger, onions, and garlic and cook for 15 minutes to caramelize the onions.

2. Add the coriander stems, spices, and 100ml of water. Pour the ingredients into the slow cooker and add the chili, passata, beans, and 400ml water. Season and cook for 5-6 hours on low.

3. When cooked, the beans should be tender, and the dal should be very thick. Add the cream and serve with a side dish of your choice.

Nutrition:

- Calories: 527
- Fat: 34g

- Carbs: 35g
- Protein: 19g

Warming Bean and Veg Soup

Preparation time: 15 minutes

Cooking time: 8 hours

Servings: 4

Ingredients:

- 2 minced garlic cloves
- 1 medium-sized potato, diced
- 2 carrots, peeled and sliced
- 2 celery stalks, diced
- A handful of frozen broad beans
- 2 tins of butter beans
- Paprika
- Worcestershire sauce
- Chili
- Salt and pepper
- Parmesan cheese
- Fresh herbs of your choice

Directions:

1. Put all the fixing except the Parmesan cheese and the fresh herbs in the slow cooker. Cook on low for 8-10 hours. Spoon onto dishes, top with Parmesan cheese and fresh herbs, and serve.

Nutrition:

- Calories: 527
- Carbohydrates: 5.2g
- Fat: 8g
- Protein: 3.7g
- Fiber: 7.4g

Slow-Cooked Baked Beans

Preparation time: 15 minutes

Cooking time: 8 hours

Servings: 8

Ingredients:

- 1 pound of beans of your choice, dried
- 1 diced medium onion
- 1/3 cup of brown sugar
- 1/3 cup of molasses
- ¼ cup of tomato sauce
- 2 tablespoons of yellow mustard
- 1 tablespoon of smoked paprika
- 1 tablespoon of Worcestershire sauce
- 1 tablespoon of cider vinegar or white balsamic vinegar
- Salt and pepper

Directions:

1. Rinse the dried beans, and pour them into the slow cooker, cover them with 2 inches of water and leave them to soak overnight.

2. The following morning, drain the water from the slow cooker and add the remaining ingredients. Put 2 and ½ cups of water, salt, and pepper to season. Cook for 8 hours on low. Spoon onto dishes and serve.

Nutrition:

- Calories: 136
- Fat: 0.2g
- Carbohydrates: 30.4g
- Protein: 3.8g

Peppers Stuffed with Black Beans & Quinoa

Preparation time: 15 minutes

Cooking time: 6 hours

Servings: 6

Ingredients:

- 6 bell peppers
- 1 cup of uncooked quinoa
- 1 can of black beans, drained
- 1 ½ cups of red enchilada sauce
- 1 teaspoon of cumin
- 1 teaspoon of chili powder
- 1 teaspoon of onion powder
- ½ a teaspoon of garlic salt
- 1 ½ cups of Pepper jack cheese, shredded, divided
- Cilantro
- Avocado
- Sour cream

Directions:

1. Cut the tops off the peppers and scrape out the insides. Combine 1 cup of cheese, spices, enchilada sauce, beans, and quinoa in a large bowl and stir thoroughly.

2. Stuff the mixture into the peppers. Pour ½ cup of water into the slow cooker. Arrange the peppers in the water. Cover and cook on high low for 6 hours.

3. Take the lid off and sprinkle the peppers with the remaining cheese, cover and cook for a few minutes to melt the cheese. Serve with avocado, sour cream, and cilantro.

Nutrition:
- Calories: 116
- Fat: 12.9g
- Carbohydrates: 59.5g
- Protein: 22.7g

Eggplant Parmesan

Preparation time: 15 minutes

Cooking time: 8 hours

Servings: 12

Ingredients:

- 4 pounds of eggplant
- 1 tablespoon of salt
- 3 large eggs
- ¼ cup of milk
- 1 ½ cup of breadcrumbs
- 3 ounces of parmesan cheese
- 2 teaspoons of Italian seasoning
- 4 cups of marinara sauce
- 16 ounces of mozzarella cheese

Directions:

1. Slice the peeled eggplant into 1/3 inch-rounds. Put the eggplant in a colander, then sprinkle each layer with salt. Let sit for 30 minutes and then rinse and pat dry.

2. Spread ½ cup of sauce on the bottom of the slow cooker. In a small bowl, whisk the milk and eggs.

3. In another small bowl, whisk the Italian seasoning, Parmesan cheese, and breadcrumbs. Soak the eggplant into the egg batter and then into the breadcrumb mixture.

4. Layer 1/3 of the slices in the slow cooker. Pour 1 cup of sauce and the mozzarella cheese over the top. Repeat twice, cover, and cook for 8 hours. Divide onto plates and serve.

Nutrition:

- Calories: 258
- Carbohydrates: 23g
- Fat: 6g
- Protein: 16g

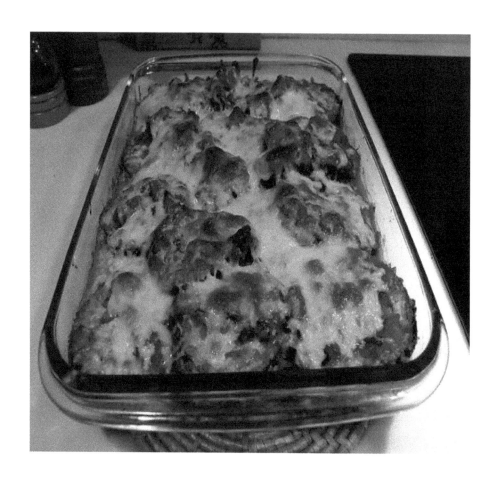

Chili Lentils and Beans

Preparation time: 15 minutes

Cooking time: 8 hours

Servings: 7

Ingredients:

- 1 finely chopped onion
- 3 garlic cloves, minced
- 1 stalk of celery, chopped
- 2 chopped bell peppers
- 1 can of diced tomatoes
- 4 cups of vegetable broth
- 1 can of water
- 1 cup of dried lentils
- 1 can of Bush's Pinto Beans
- 2 tablespoons of chili powder
- 2 teaspoons of cumin
- 1 tablespoon of oregano

Directions:

1. Put all of the fixings into the slow cooker and cook for 8 hours on low. Serve with a combination of cilantro, green onion, avocado, sour cream, plain Greek Yogurt, and shredded cheese.

Nutrition:

- Calories: 192
- Carbs: 25g
- Fat: 2g
- Protein: 13g

Butternut Macaroni Squash

Preparation time: 15 minutes

Cooking time: 8 hours

Servings: 5

Ingredients:

- 1 ½ cups of butternut squash, cubed
- ½ cup of chopped tomatoes
- 1 ½ cups of water
- 2 minced garlic cloves
- A handful of fresh thyme, finely chopped
- A handful of fresh rosemary, finely chopped
- ¼ cup of nutritional yeast
- 1 cup of non-dairy milk
- 1 ½ cups of whole wheat macaroni
- Salt and pepper

Directions:

1. Add the butternut squash, diced tomatoes, water, garlic, thyme, and rosemary to the slow cooker. Cover and cook on low within 7-9 hours.

2.   Transfer the ingredients from the slow cooker into a food processor and add the nutritional yeast, half a cup of non-dairy milk, and blend.

3.   Pour the ingredients back into the slow cooker, add the macaroni, cover, and cook for a further 20 minutes on high. Stir, cook for a further 25 minutes and add salt and pepper to taste. Spoon onto dishes and serve.

Nutrition:

- Calories: 187
- Fat: 2g
- Carbohydrates: 35g
- Protein: 8g

Veggie Pot Pie

Preparation time: 15 minutes

Cooking time: 4 hours

Servings: 6

Ingredients:

- 6-7 cups of chopped veggies of your choice
- ½ cup of diced onions
- 4 minced garlic cloves
- Fresh thyme, finely chopped
- ½ cup of flour
- 2 cups of chicken broth
- ¼ cup of cornstarch
- ¼ cup of heavy cream
- Salt and pepper
- 1 thawed frozen puff pastry sheet
- 2 tablespoons of butter

Directions:

1. Put the chopped veggies in the slow cooker, put the garlic and onions. Add the flour. Add the broth and stir until everything is well blended. Cover and cook for 3-4 hours on high.

2. In a small bowl, combine the cornstarch and ¼ cup of water and whisk thoroughly. Put the cornstarch mix in the slow cooker.

3. Add the cream, cover, and continue to cook until the mixture thickens approximately 15 minutes. Transfer the vegetable mixture into a baking dish.

4. Lay the puff pastry over the top. Melt the butter and brush it over the top of the pastry. Bake at 350 degrees for 10 minutes until the pastry turns fluffy and golden. Divide onto dishes and serve.

Nutrition:

- Calories: 325
- Fat: 0.8g
- Protein: 4.5g
- Carbohydrates: 6.7g

Barbecue Beef Stew

Preparation time: 15 minutes

Cooking time: 8 hours

Servings: 6

Ingredients:

¾ cup of each:

- Homemade tomato paste
- Balsamic vinegar
- ½ tsp black pepper

1 teaspoon of each:

- Smoked paprika
- Kosher salt
- Garlic powder
- 2 tbsp. sweetener

For the Stew:

- 1 tsp kosher salt
- 2 lb. extra-lean stew beef meat/boneless chuck roast
- 1 tbsp. olive oil
- ½ t. black pepper
- 2 tbsp. cold tap water
- 1 tbsp cornstarch or ½ t. konjac flour

- Also Needed: 14-inch skillet

Directions:

1. Chop the meat into one-inch pieces, and season it with pepper and salt. Combine the barbecue sauce ingredients.

2. Prepare the skillet by adding half of the oil using the med-high setting for three minutes. Add half of the beef and cook for about five minutes.

3. Place in the slow cooker. Add the rest of the oil and cook the second half of beef and add it also. Empty the sauce over the prepared meat and stir. Place the top on the pot and cook for 7 ½ hours on low.

4. Whisk in the cornstarch and water in a dish until smooth. Empty it into the beef juices. Set the slow cooker on high for 30 minutes. When thickened to your liking, serve, and enjoy.

Nutrition:

- Calories: 445
- Carbs: 10g
- Protein: 30g
- Fat: 29g

Beef Stew with Tomatoes

Preparation time: 15 minutes

Cooking time: 8 hours

Servings: 6

Ingredients:

- 1 pkg. (5lbs.) stew beef
- 2 cans chili-ready diced tomatoes (14.5oz.) - organic
- 2 tsp hot sauce
- 1 cup of beef broth
- 1 tbsp. of each:
- Chili mix (pre-packaged)
- Worcestershire sauce
- Salt to taste

Directions:

1. Warm up the slow cooker in the high setting. Add the stewing beef, tomatoes, hot sauce, broth, Worcestershire sauce, chili mix, and salt in the slow cooker.

2. Set the timer for six hours. Break the meat apart and continue cooking for another two hours. Sprinkle with a pinch of salt to taste when ready to serve.

Nutrition:

- Calories: 222
- Carbs: 9g
- Fat: 7g
- Protein: 27g

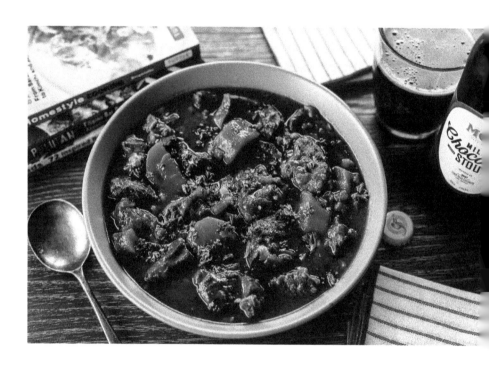

Chicken Stew

Preparation time: 15 minutes

Cooking time: 2 hours

Servings: 4

Ingredients:

- 1 pkg. (28oz.) skinless & deboned chicken thighs
- 2 celery sticks, diced
- ½ cup diced of each:
- Onion
- 2 medium carrots – approx.
- 2 cup of chicken stock
- ½ tsp dried rosemary/1 fresh sprig
- 3 minced garlic cloves
- Pepper and salt to taste
- ½ tsp dried oregano
- ¼ tsp dried thyme
- ½ cup of heavy cream
- 1 cup of fresh spinach
- Xanthan gum as desired (start at 1/8 tsp)
- Recommended: 3-quart or larger slow cooker

Directions:

1. Dice the chicken into one-inch chunks. Remove the skin, and finely dice the carrots and celery. Add the veggies and chicken to the slow cooker.

2. Pour in the stock, thyme, oregano, rosemary, and garlic in the cooker. Toss in the pepper and salt. Mix in the heavy cream and spinach leaves.

3. Add the xanthan gum to thicken the juices, and simmer another ten minutes. Set the cooker on high for two hours or low setting for four hours. When it's done, enjoy.

Nutrition:

- Calories: 228
- Carbs: 6g
- Fat: 11g
- Protein: 23g

Hare Stew

Preparation time: 15 minutes

Cooking time: 5 hours

Servings: 6

Ingredients:

- ½ lb. uncured organic bacon/smoked pork belly
- 1 whole rabbit/hare (3lb.) cut into pieces
- 2 tbsp. butter
- 2 cups of dry white wine
- 1 large of each:
- Sweet onion
- Sprig of rosemary
- 1 tsp whole peppercorn
- 2 bay leaves
- 2 tbsp. Celtic sea salt

Directions:

1. Cut the pork belly into one-inch bites. Place them in a heated skillet along with the butter. Thinly slice the onion, and toss it in.

2. Continue cooking slowly for approximately five minutes and remove the onion (leaving the grease in the skillet).

Arrange the prepared meat bites in the pan, and continue cooking using the high setting until browned.

3. Pour in the wine, then simmer for two more minutes. Add all the fixings into the slow cooker. Shake in the rosemary, salt, bay leaves, and peppercorn. Select the low setting for five hours. When done, serve, and enjoy.

Nutrition:

- Calories: 517
- Protein: 36g
- Carbs: 2g
- Fat: 32

Herb Chicken & Mushroom Stew

Preparation time: 15 minutes

Cooking time: 4 hours

Servings: 5

Ingredients:

- 1lb. raw chicken tenders
- 24oz. whole white button mushrooms

½ tsp dried of each:

- Oregano
- Basil
- 3 garlic cloves
- ¼ tsp dried thyme
- 1 cup of chicken broth
- 2 bay leaves
- Pepper
- Salt
- 2 tbsp. butter
- ¼ cup of heavy whipping cream
- 8 bacon slices – chopped & cooked
- ¼ cup of freshly chopped parsley

Directions:

1. Cut the stems on the larger mushrooms and wash. Dice into bite-sized pieces and place them in the slow cooker.

2. Arrange the chicken in the pot along with the spices (garlic, basil thyme, oregano, and bay leaves) and broth. Give it a shake of the pepper and salt.

3. Set the timer for three to four hours using the low-temperature setting. Combine the butter and whipping cream. Jazz it up with some salt and pepper to your liking. Serve with the parsley and bacon bits.

Nutrition:

- Calories: 297.2
- Carbs: 4.42g
- Fat: 17.5g
- Protein: 29.99g

Hungarian Beef Goulash

Preparation time: 15 minutes

Cooking time: 4 hours

Servings: 8

Ingredients:

- 2 lb. beef stew meat – cubed
- 2 garlic cloves
- 1 cup of onion – chopped
- 1 tsp salt

2 tbsp. of each:

- Hungarian paprika
- Butter/bacon grease
- ½ tsp of each:
- Caraway seeds
- Pepper
- 2 sliced celery stalks
- 1 yellow/green chopped bell pepper
- 2 cup of cubed daikon radishes
- 1 can (15oz.) diced tomatoes
- 1 ½ cup of beef/chicken broth
- 1 bay leaf

Directions:

1. Prepare a skillet with the butter using the medium heat setting until it's melted. Stir in the onions and cook until translucent. Toss in the paprika and garlic, stirring for another minute.

2. Add the beef, and sprinkle with the pepper, salt, and caraway seeds into the cooker. Fold in the peppers, radish, celery, broth, bay leaf, and tomatoes.

3. Mix thoroughly and prepare using the low setting for six hours. You can also choose four hours using the high setting. Serve!

Nutrition:

- Calories: 345
- Carbs: 5.52g
- Fat: 23.88g
- Protein: 23.84g

Vegetable Beef Stew

Preparation time : 15 minutes

Cooking time: 7 hours

Servings: 10

Ingredients :

- 1 lb. boneless beef braising steaks
- 1 ½ tsp salt – ex. pink Himalayan
- Freshly ground black pepper
- ½ cup of tallow/lard/ghee
- 1 medium white onion
- 4 garlic cloves
- 1 cup of vegetable stock/broth/water
- 2 tbsp. ground cumin

1 tsp of each:

- Turmeric powder
- Ground coriander seeds
- Paprika
- Chili powder
- Ground ginger
- 2 cinnamon sticks
- 1 can (14.1oz.) unsweetened tomatoes – chopped
- 4-5 medium zucchini

- 2 bay leaves
- 1 medium rutabaga – 1.3 lb.
- Suggested: 6-quart slow cooker

Directions:

1. Warm up the cooker on the high setting. Dry the liquids off the steaks with a paper towel. Give the meat a shake of the salt and pepper.

2. Sear the steaks in a skillet with ¼ cup of the butter/ghee. Add to the slow cooker. Peel and dice the garlic and onion. Toss it into the pan with the rest of the ghee.

3. Pour in the tomatoes, turmeric, coriander seeds, chili powder, broth, cumin, and paprika. Gently combine and add to the slow cooker on top of the meat.

4. Put the bay leaves and cinnamon sticks in the cooker. Put the top on the pot. Cook for three hours, and then add the rutabaga on the side of the meat.

5. Cook another hour and add the diced zucchini. Mix and remove the cinnamon sticks and bay leaves when done. Cook for two additional hours. If desired, sprinkle with more pepper and salt. Top it off with some of the fresh herbs and enjoy.

Nutrition:

- Calories: 533

- Carbs: 9.1g
- Fat: 39.5g
- Protein: 31.9g

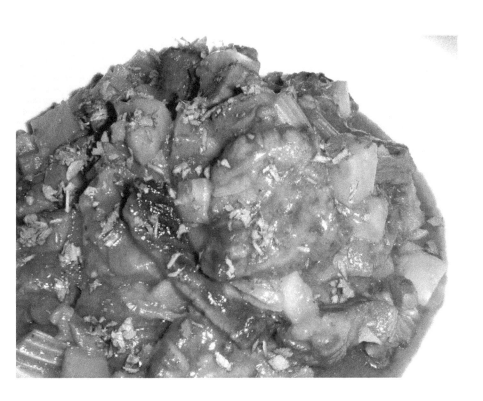

Bone Broth

Preparation time: 15 minutes

Cooking time: 6 hours

Servings: 8

Ingredients:

- 3 ½ lb. assorted mixed bones – ex. marrow bones, chicken feet, or your choice
- 1 tbsp. pink Himalayan salt

1 medium of each:

- Parsnip
- White onion – skin on
- 5 peeled garlic cloves
- 2 mediums of each:
- Celery stalks
- Carrots
- 2 tbsp. apple cider vinegar or lemon juice
- 8 cups of water

Directions:

1. Peel and slice the vegetables with roots into 1/3-inch pieces. Slice the onion in half. Chop the celery into thirds. Add the bay leaves into the slow cooker.

2. Toss in the chosen bones (can also be pork). Pour the water up to ¾ capacity—along with the juice/vinegar and bay leaves. Sprinkle with the salt.

3. Secure the lid. Choose either low for ten hours or high six hours. You can simmer up to 48 hours. Remove the bits of veggies using a strainer. Set the bones aside to chill. Shred the meat and use it as desired.

4. Refrigerate the broth overnight. Scrape away the tallow (greasy layer) if desired. Use within five days or freeze. You can also keep it in the canning jars for up to 45 days.

Nutrition:

- Calories: 72
- Fat: 6g
- Carbs: 0.7g
- Protein: 3.6g

Cabbage & Ground Beef Soup

Preparation time: 15 minutes

Cooking time: 3 hours

Servings: 4

Ingredients:

- 2 tbsp. olive oil

½ cup chopped of each:

- Shallots
- Onions
- 2 minced garlic cloves
- 2 lb. ground beef
- 1 tsp each of:
- Salt
- Pepper
- Dried parsley
- ½ tsp dried oregano
- 16oz. marinara sauce
- 2 cups of riced cauliflower – ½ head
- 5 cups of low-sodium beef broth
- 8 cup of sliced cabbage – 1 large

Directions:

1. In a skillet on the med-high heat setting, warm up the oil. When hot, stir in the garlic, shallots, and onions. Sauté until softened. Stir in the beef—cooking until pink is gone.

2. Toss in the seasonings and marinara sauce. Fold in the riced cauliflower and stir well. Pour the fixings into the slow cooker.

3. Empty in the beef broth and cabbage. Stir. Prepare to cook for six hours on low or three on the high setting. When done, have a seat and enjoy it.

Nutrition:

- Calories: 312
- Carbs: 9.8g
- Fat: 15.2g
- Protein: 31.1g

Cheesy Mexican Chicken Soup

Preparation time: 15 minutes

Cooking time: 4 hours

Servings: 6

Ingredients:

- 1 ½ lb. chicken thighs
- 15oz. chicken broth
- 15 ½oz. chunky salsa – ex. Tostitos
- 8oz. Pepper Jack/Monterey cheese

Directions:

1. Cut out any bones and remove the fat from the chicken. Arrange them in the slow cooker. Mix in the rest of the fixings. Set the cooker using the low setting for six to eight hours or three to four on the high setting.

2. When the time is up, remove and shred the chicken. Put it back in the cooker to mingle with the juices for a minute or so. Stir and serve right out of the slow cooker.

Nutrition:

- Calories: 400
- Carbs: 5.1g
- Fat: 22.8g

- Protein: 28g

Chicken & Bacon Chowder

Preparation time: 15 minutes

Cooking time: 8 hours

Servings: 8

Ingredients:

- 1 trimmed – sliced leek
- 6oz. sliced cremini mushrooms
- 1 finely chopped shallot
- 1 med. thinly sliced sweet onion
- 4 minced garlic cloves
- 4 tbsp. butter – divided
- 2 diced celery ribs
- 2 cups of chicken stock – divided
- 1 lb. chicken breasts
- 1 pkg. (8oz.) cream cheese
- 1 lb. bacon – crispy & crumbled
- 1 cup of heavy cream

1 tsp of each:

- Sea salt
- Dried thyme
- Black pepper
- Garlic powder

Directions:

1. Using the low setting for one hour, add the shallot, garlic, leek, mushrooms, celery, onions, one cup of the chicken stock, black pepper, sea salt, and two tablespoons butter to the slow cooker. Secure the lid.

2. In a skillet, sear the chicken breasts over the med-high setting on the stovetop using the rest of the butter. It should take approximately five minutes per side—making sure they are browned evenly. Set aside on a platter.

3. Deglaze the pan with the rest of the stock using a rubber spatula. Add the chicken to the slow cooker and pour in the cream, garlic powder, thyme, and cream cheese. Combine the mixture until the chunks of cheese are consumed in the mixture.

4. After the chicken has cooled down, cut it into cubes, and toss it into the cooker along with the bacon. Mix well. Cover and simmer for six to eight hours (low). When done, serve, and enjoy.

Nutrition:

- Calories: 355
- Carbs: 5.75g
- Fat: 28g
- Protein: 21g

Kale & Chicken Soup

Preparation time: 15 minutes

Cooking time: 6 hours

Servings : 6

Ingredients:

- 2lb. chicken thighs/breast meat
- 1/3 cup of onion
- ½ cup (+) 1 tbsp. olive oil
- 14oz. chicken broth
- 32oz. chicken stock
- 5oz. baby kale leaves
- Salt & pepper to taste
- ¼ cup of lemon juice

Also Needed:

- Large skillet
- Blender

Directions:

1. Remove all skin, including bones, from the chicken. Dice the onions. Heat-up one tbsp of the oil in a frying pan (med. heat). Sprinkle the pepper and salt on the chicken. Toss it into the pan.

2. Lower the temperature to med-low and cover. Continue cooking the chicken until it reaches the internal temperature of 165°F (approximately 15 minutes).

3. Shred your cooked chicken, and add it to the slow cooker. Use the blender to combine the rest of the oil, onion, and chicken broth.

4. Scrape it into the cooker. Stir in the rest of the ingredients and cover. Prepare for 6 hours. Stir a few times during the final cycle. Serve and enjoy.

Nutrition:

- Calories: 261
- Carbs: 2g
- Protein: 14.1g
- Fat: 21g

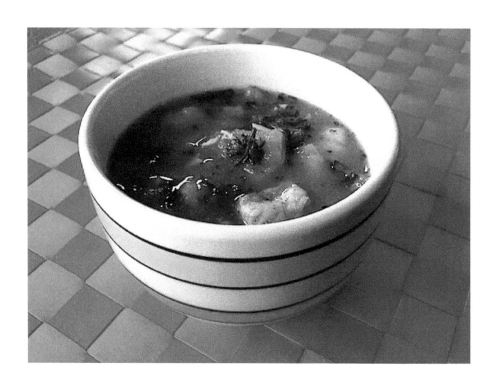

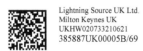
Lightning Source UK Ltd.
Milton Keynes UK
UKHW020733210621
385887UK00005B/69